Acknowledgements

The authors are very grateful to the Department of Medical Photography at St Mary's Hospital, London, and the Departments of Medical Illustration at St Bartholomew's Hospital, London and Ipswich Hospital, for their help in obtaining material for the book. Thanks also to Mr J. Wright (Figs 27, 44, 54 and 75), Dr A. Choy (Figs 25, 30 and 34), Dr T. Lissauer (Figs 94, 126 and 138), Mr D. Archer (Figs 83 and 149), Mr N. Breach (Fig. 9), Mr D. Davies (Fig. 145), Mr J. Eyre (Fig. 104), Dr A. Forge (Fig. 46), Dr J. M. Henk (Fig. 108), Mr C. M. Bailey (Fig. 91) and Mr P. Rhys-Evans (Fig. 109). The authors particularly appreciate the generosity of Professor Michael Hawke in offering them the use of some of his excellent tele-otoscopic pictures (Figs 5, 11, 13, 19, 23 and 29). Finally, the authors wish to express their gratitude to the patients appearing in this book, without whose cooperation this work would not have been possible.

London   N.D.S.
1994   R.Y.

Contents

1 / **Congenital ear disease**

External ear

Clinical features The pinna may be absent or rudimentary (microtia) (Fig. 1). Failure of obliteration of the first branchial cleft results in a congenital sinus usually found in front of the helix or tragus (Fig. 2) which may become a site of infection requiring its excision. Accessory auricles can occur adjacent to a normally placed pinna (Fig. 3).

Middle ear

Clinical features Ossicular chain defects often occur in association with atresia of the external auditory canal. Treacher-Collins syndrome consists of middle and external ear malformation with abnormal facial bone development.

Management Bone anchored hearing aids and auricular prostheses (Fig. 4) have greatly improved the treatment of these conditions, particularly in bilateral cases. With this technique prostheses are secured directly to the bones of the skull via osseo-integrated screws passing through the skin.

Inner ear

Congenital defects of the inner ear usually result in severe sensorineural deafness. These disorders may have an hereditary basis. Damage to the inner ear can also be caused by events during pregnancy and the perinatal period; these include infections, particularly maternal rubella and syphilis, haemolytic disease of the newborn and fetal anoxia during birth.

Management In the management of congenital ear disease it is vital that deafness, if present, is detected at an early stage so that treatment is instituted allowing optimum language development during early childhood.

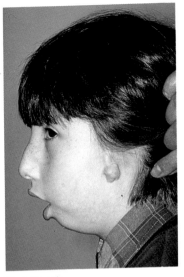

Fig. 1 Microtia.

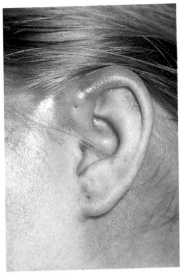

Fig. 2 Preauricular sinus.

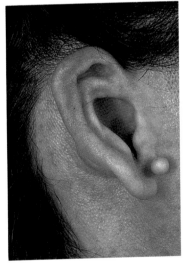

Fig. 3 Accessory auricles.

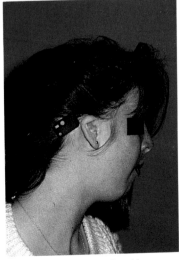

Fig. 4 Bone anchored hearing aid.

2 / External ear trauma

Foreign bodies

Clinical features
Foreign bodies are most commonly found in children, e.g. beads, cotton wool buds (Fig. 5). If deeply inserted into the external ear canal they may cause tympanic membrane perforation (Fig. 6).

Management
Removal of foreign bodies may require a general anaesthetic. Most traumatic tympanic membrane perforations heal spontaneously.

Cauliflower ear

Clinical features
Blunt trauma to the pinna may produce a subperichondrial haematoma (Fig. 7). Devoid of its blood supply the cartilage necroses and is replaced by fibrous tissue resulting in an ugly cosmetic deformity (Fig. 8).

Management
Early drainage of the haematoma usually prevents any deformity.

Perichondritis

Perichondritis may result from open trauma, which may be surgical, involving the cartilage of the pinna or auditory meatus. Occasionally complicates a severe otitis externa.

Clinical features
Presents as a generalised red, painful and tender swelling of the pinna and oedema may also stenose the meatus. A severe facial cellulitis and necrosis of the cartilage may develop.

Management
Treatment is with antibiotics and surgical drainage of any abscess.

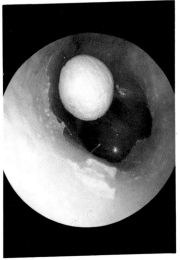

Fig. 5 Foreign body in the external canal.

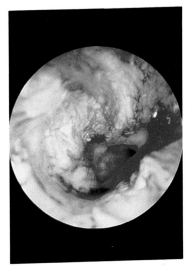

Fig. 6 Traumatic perforation.

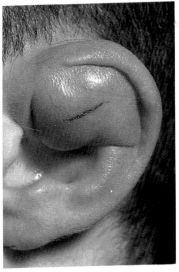

Fig. 7 Subperichondrial haematoma due to trauma.

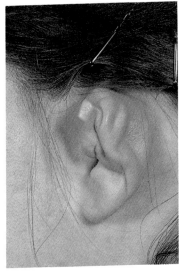

Fig. 8 Cauliflower ear.

3 / Tumours of the pinna and external auditory meatus

Malignant tumours

Basal cell carcinomas, squamous cell carcinomas (Fig. 9) and malignant melanomas occur on the skin of the pinna. Exposure to sunlight over a long period is a major risk factor.

Clinical features Initially small superficial lesions progressing to deep ulceration in advanced cases. Squamous carcinomas and malignant melanomas metastasize to regional cervical lymph nodes.

Management Treated by surgical excision, although radiotherapy is an alternative for basal and squamous carcinomas. Involvement of cartilage renders the tumour less radiosensitive.

Benign tumours

Osteoma of the external auditory meatus is most common.

Aetiology Osteomas are associated with repeated exposure of the external auditory meatus to cold water as in swimming and diving.

Clinical features Solitary or multiple, osteomas present as smooth swellings on the wall of the bony meatus (Fig. 10). They are often asymptomatic, but if the lumen of the meatus is occluded, retention of wax, otitis externa or hearing loss may occur.

Management None if asymptomatic. If recurrent otitis externa occurs osteomas may be surgically reduced.

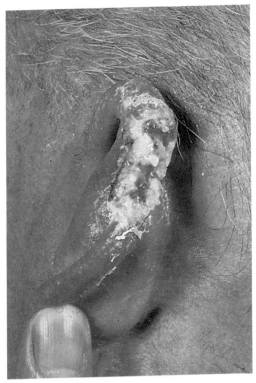

Fig. 9 Squamous carcinoma of the pinna.

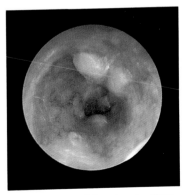

Fig. 10 Osteomas of the external auditory canal.

4 / Otitis externa

Definition   Inflammation of the skin of the external auditory meatus.

Aetiology   It is caused by either primary infection or contact sensitivity to topically applied substances such as cosmetics or antibiotics. Gram-negative organisms (e.g. *Proteus, Pseudomonas*) and fungi (e.g. *Aspergillus*) are often found. Precipitating factors include impacted cerumen, local trauma, middle ear discharge through a tympanic membrane perforation, swimming and skin conditions such as psoriasis and seborrhoeic dermatitis.

Clinical features   Presents as otalgia, otorrhoea and deafness. The skin of the external auditory meatus is oedematous and inflamed (Figs 11 & 12). The meatus may be occluded with discharge and in fungal infections hypae may be seen (Fig. 13). Traction on the pinna increases the otalgia, a sign not found in inflammatory conditions of the middle ear.

Management   Debris must be removed from the meatus, either by dry mopping, or suction aided by the use of an operating microscope. A swab of the meatus is taken for bacteriology prior to the instillation of drops containing an antibiotic and steroid mixture. If the meatus is totally occluded an impregnated gauze wick may be inserted. In severe cases with cellulitis spreading onto the pinna (Fig. 14) systemic antibiotics are also needed.

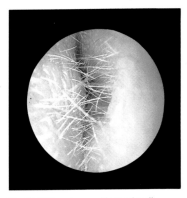

Fig. 11 Otitis externa with canal wall oedema.

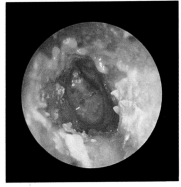

Fig. 12 Bacterial otitis externa.

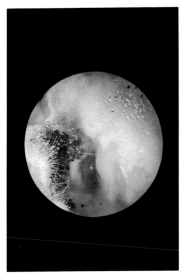

Fig. 13 Fungal otitis externa.

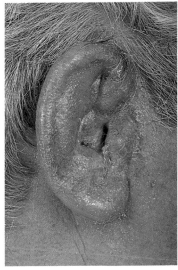

Fig. 14 Cellulitis of the pinna secondary to otitis externa.

Furunculosis of the external auditory meatus

Staphylococcal infection of hair follicles found in the lateral part of the meatus.

Clinical features   Presents as severe otalgia exacerbated by traction on the pinna, with deafness if the meatus becomes occluded. The furuncle is often visible.

Management   Most furuncles rupture spontaneously. Ribbon gauze impregnated with glycerin/ichthammol may be inserted daily into the meatus (Fig. 15). Systemic flucloxacillin and analgesics are also needed.

Malignant otitis externa

A potentially fatal *Pseudomonas* infection of the external auditory meatus. It occurs in elderly diabetics with spread to the skull base.

Clinical features   Presents as severe otalgia, otorrhoea and deafness with progression to cranial nerve palsies (VII, IX, X, XI, XII) in advanced cases.

Management   Treatment is by local surgery, usually mastoidectomy, combined with a prolonged course of specific anti-pseudomonal antibiotics. Skull base involvement and its response to treatment may be assessed by radioisotope scanning (Fig. 16).

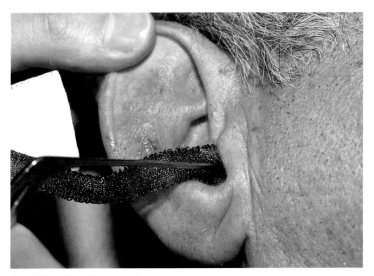

Fig. 15 Glycerin and ichthammol wick insertion.

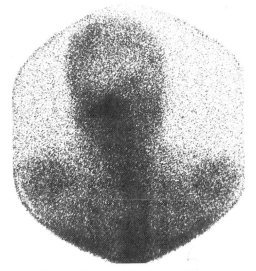

Fig. 16 Gallium scan in malignant otitis externa: increased uptake at petrous apex.

5 / Local conditions of the tympanic membrane

Bullous myringitis

Aetiology An influenza virus infection of the tympanic membrane and deep external meatus, often associated with an acute otitis media.

Clinical features Presents as otalgia, deafness and serosanguinous otorrhoea. Haemorrhagic bullae are seen on otoscopy (Fig. 17). Secondary bacterial infection can occur with purulent otorrhoea leading to otitis externa.

Management Treat with analgesics; local and systemic antibiotics for secondary bacterial infection.

Tympanosclerosis

Aetiology Deposits of collagen beneath the mucosa of the tympanic membrane and middle ear following otitis media or middle ear surgery, particularly grommet insertion.

Clinical features Tympanosclerosis is mostly asymptomatic. Deposits are visible as white 'chalk patches' in the tympanic membrane (Fig. 18). Middle ear deposits may cause conductive deafness by ossicular fixation.

Management None if asymptomatic. Ossiculoplasty may be required for conductive deafness.

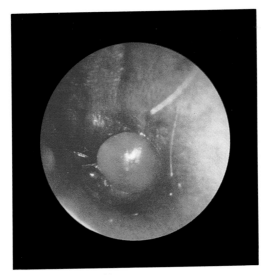

Fig. 17 Bullous myringitis.

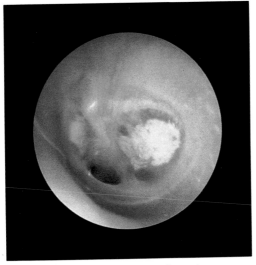

Fig. 18 Tympanosclerosis of the tympanic membrane.

6 / Middle ear effusions

Aetiology   Middle ear effusion is often associated with eustachian tube obstruction, either acute during upper respiratory infections or chronic as in childhood adenoid hypertrophy. In adults middle ear effusions may result from eustachian tube obstruction by a nasopharyngeal neoplasm. Changes in atmospheric pressure occurring during airflight and diving may also result in effusions—otitic barotrauma.

Incidence   Middle ear effusion is a common paediatric problem, particularly in the 4–7 age group.

Clinical features   On otoscopy the tympanic membrane is dull with a loss of light reflex (Fig. 19). Small vessels are often seen radiating from the handle of the malleus and occasionally a fluid level is seen (Fig. 20). Deafness in children may lead to poor language development and educational performance. Diagnosis may be confirmed by impedance audiometry in which the compliance of the tympanic membrane is measured in response to pressure changes in the external auditory meatus.

Management   **Medical treatment** consists of the use of topical and systemic decongestants.

Surgical treatment consists of myringotomy and insertion of a ventilation tube into the affected tympanic membrane (Figs 21 & 22). Children may also require an adenoidectomy whilst in adults a nasopharyngeal tumour must be excluded.

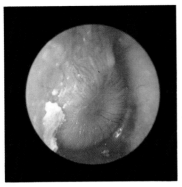

Fig. 19 'Glue' ear.

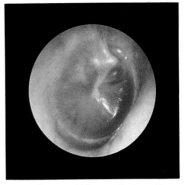

Fig. 20 Serous middle ear effusion with fluid level.

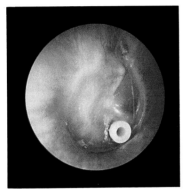

Fig. 21 Grommet in situ.

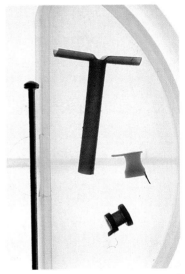

Fig. 22 Types of ventilation tubes: Goode T tube, Shah and Sheppard grommets (top to bottom).

7 / Suppurative otitis media

Acute otitis media

Aetiology Acute infection of the middle ear cleft, common in young children. This usually occurs as part of an upper respiratory tract infection with *Haemophilus influenzae* and *Pneumococcus* being the most common pathogens.

Clinical features Presents as severe otalgia and deafness. The tympanic membrane is red and bulging (Fig. 23). Rupture may occur leading to purulent otorrhoea.

Management Treat with oral antibiotic therapy (amoxycillin, cotrimoxazole or erythromycin) and adequate analgesia.

Acute mastoiditis

Aetiology Acute mastoiditis may complicate acute otitis media. Infection of the mastoid air cell system occurs.

Clinical features Worsening of otalgia with tenderness over the mastoid antrum presents. The external meatus may be narrowed by oedema of the posterior-superior wall. In advanced cases a subperiosteal abscess may push the ear forward (Fig. 24). Diagnosis is confirmed by opacity of the mastoid cells on X-ray.

Management Initially high dose parenteral antibiotic therapy is required, although in cases which fail to respond to antibiotics, or in which a subperiosteal abscess has formed, surgical drainage via a cortical mastoidectomy is required.

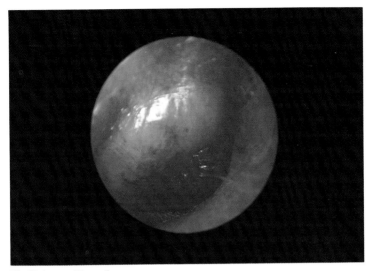

Fig. 23 Acute otitis media.

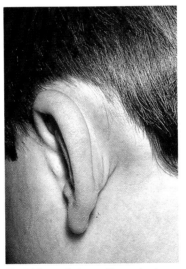

Fig. 24 Postauricular swelling and redness in acute mastoiditis.

Chronic otitis media

Aetiology Chronic inflammation of the middle ear cleft is usually associated with a perforation of the tympanic membrane. Perforations usually result from previous episodes of acute otitis media when the membrane fails to heal following rupture, but can be due to direct or indirect trauma. In children, perforations can persist following extrusion of ventilation tubes from the tympanic membrane. Organisms can reach the middle ear from the eustachian tube or from the external meatus. Chronic middle ear infection is also associated with ossicular damage with the incudo-stapedial joint being the most commonly affected linkage.

Clinical features A *central perforation* in the pars tensa part of the membrane (Figs 25 & 26) is associated with recurrent otorrhoea and conductive deafness. This type of perforation is regarded as 'safe' as neurological complications are rare. An *attic or marginal perforation* (Fig. 27) can be associated with the development of a cholesteatoma and is regarded as 'unsafe'.

Management Cases of central perforation should be kept dry. If recurrent otorrhoea occurs ear drops containing a mixture of steroid and antibiotic are used and attention paid to possible sources of infection in the nasopharynx, nose and paranasal sinuses. A dry perforation can be repaired by myringoplasty. Traumatic central perforations usually heal spontaneously.

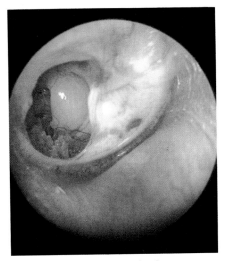

Fig. 25 Dry posterior central perforation.

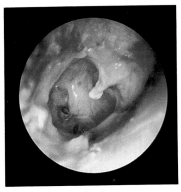

Fig. 26 Subtotal perforation.

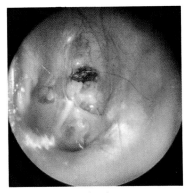

Fig. 27 Dry attic perforation.

8 / Cholesteatoma

A ball of keratinizing stratified squamous epithelium in the middle ear cleft or mastoid which enlarges and can destroy or erode local structures. It is a feature of the 'unsafe' type of chronic middle ear disease.

Aetiology   The most widely accepted theory of its development is the immigration-retraction pocket theory: in response to eustachian tube obstruction and negative middle ear pressure an inward retraction of the tympanic membrane occurs, usually in the attic region. Desquamated epithelium normally shed from the membrane into the meatus collects in the pocket, the continued enlargement of which results in the formation of a cholesteatoma sac. Congenital cholesteatoma is very rare (Fig. 28) and results from congenital squamous cell rests within the temporal bone.

Clinical features   Presents as progressive conductive hearing loss with purulent, and often offensive, otorrhoea. Pain or vertigo due to bony erosion may also occur. Otoscopy reveals a retraction pocket or perforation in the attic or posterior marginal region of the tympanic membrane (Fig. 29) with flaky white debris visible in the defect. Nystagmus and other evidence of neurological involvement should be sought.

Management   Radical mastoidectomy involves removal of the cholesteatoma, middle ear structures and bone of the bony external meatus, producing a smooth exteriorised mastoid cavity accessible for inspection. The operation may be modified in order to conserve hearing by retaining part of the ossicular chain and tympanic membrane (Fig. 30).

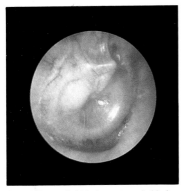

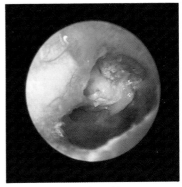

Fig. 28 Congenital cholesteatoma behind an intact tympanic membrane.

Fig. 29 Attic perforation with cholesteatoma.

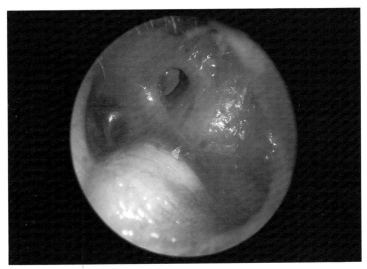

Fig. 30 Healed right modified radical mastoidectomy cavity.

9 / Complications of suppurative otitis media

Facial nerve paralysis

Aetiology Pressure by cholesteatoma on the facial nerve in the middle ear or mastoid.

Clinical features Presents as partial or complete lower motor neurone facial paralysis (Fig. 31) with evidence of chronic middle ear disease on otoscopy.

Management Treatment is by immediate surgical decompression of the facial nerve via a mastoidectomy operation.

Suppurative labyrinthitis

Aetiology Follows erosion of the bony labyrinth most commonly over the lateral semicircular canal. In the early stages compression of the air in the external meatus causes vertigo from mechanical stimulation of the labyrinth (Fistula test). Later purulent infection in the inner ear causes severe vertigo and sensorineural deafness.

Management Treatment is by intravenous antibiotics and eradication of cholesteatoma via mastoidectomy.

Gradenigo's syndrome

Otorrhoea is associated with pain behind the eye and diplopia, caused by fifth and sixth nerve irritation resulting from air cell infection at the petrous apex (Fig. 32).

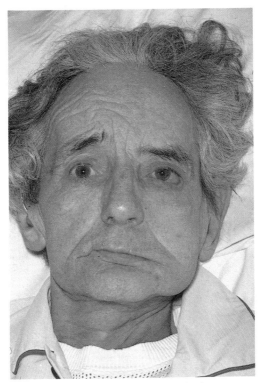

Fig. 31 Complete lower motor neurone facial palsy.

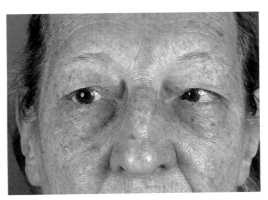

Fig. 32 Gradenigo's syndrome: patient looking to right.

Intracranial spread of organisms may occur via the middle ear, by thrombophlebitis or by penetration of the dura of the middle or posterior cranial fossae.

Meningitis

Clinical features
Presents as headache, neck stiffness and photophobia. Lumbar puncture confirms the diagnosis.
Pneumococcus and *Haemophilus influenzae* are common pathogens.

Management
Treatment is by intravenous antibiotics followed by mastoidectomy once the meningitis has resolved.

Venous sinus thrombosis

Follows spread of middle ear and mastoid infection through the bone over the sigmoid sinus.

Clinical features
Presents as headache, pyrexia and rigors. Extension of thrombus to the superior sagittal sinus leads to CSF outflow obstruction—otitic hydrocephalus.

Management
Treatment is by intravenous antibiotics and mastoidectomy, during which infected thrombus may need to be removed from the sigmoid sinus lumen.

Intracranial abscess

Extradural, subdural and cerebral abscesses occur. Infection spreads into the middle and posterior cranial fossae leading to temporal lobe and cerebellar abscesses respectively. Diagnosis is by CT scan (Fig. 33) and treatment by neurosurgical drainage.

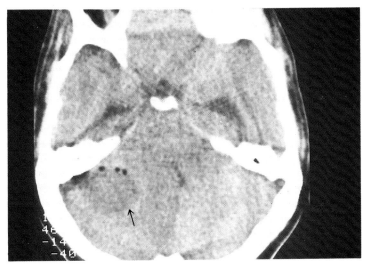

Fig. 33 Otogenic cerebellar abscess on CT scan.

10 / Otosclerosis

A disease primarily of the bone of the otic capsule which causes a conductive hearing loss, usually because of stapes fixation. A sensorineural deafness may occur in later stages.

Incidence The disease is usually bilateral and presents between the ages of 15 and 45 years. Tinnitus is common and 25% of patients have positional vertigo. 70% have family history of otosclerosis.

Clinical features Examination of the tympanic membrane is usually normal, the pink drum (Schwartze sign) being rare and indicative of active disease (Fig. 34). In the early stages the audiogram shows a pure conductive loss, frequently with a Cahart's notch at 2000 Hz (Fig. 35).

Management An air conduction hearing aid is frequently very successful for the patient. In the stapedectomy operation the stapes arch is replaced by a piston, usually made of teflon (Fig. 36). Stapedectomy will produce excellent improvement in hearing level in the majority of cases, although profound deafness and vertigo are occasional complications.

A rare variant is seen in association with osteogenesis imperfecta (van der Hoeve syndrome), these patients being recognised by their blue sclera. Stapedectomy is less successful in these cases.

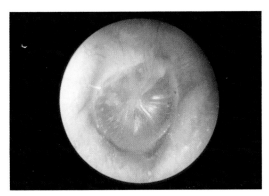

Fig. 34 Schwartze sign: flamingo pink flush behind tympanic membrane.

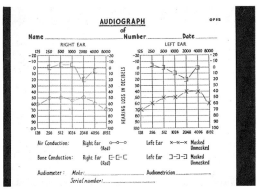

Fig. 35 Pure tone audiogram with bilateral Cahart's notches.

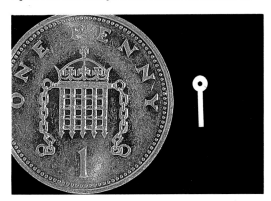

Fig. 36 Teflon stapes prosthesis.

11 / Middle ear microsurgery

Myringoplasty

Central perforations may be repaired when accompanied by deafness or recurrent middle ear infections or when an intact tympanic membrane is required for swimming or as a condition of employment. Fascia overlying the temporalis muscle is usually used (Fig. 37) and may be placed medial (underlay) or lateral (onlay) to the perforation.

Ossiculoplasty

Performed for conductive deafness where the ossicular chain has been interrupted by chronic infection, trauma or congenital deformity. Replacement ossicles may be constructed from natural or synthetic materials. Bone is the favoured material, where possible the patient's own incus remnant is remodelled and transposed.

Eradication of mastoid disease—mastoidectomy

Performed for acute mastoiditis failing to respond to high dose antibiotics, otorrhoea due to chronic mastoid infection, and middle ear and mastoid cholesteatoma.

Cortical mastoidectomy involves exenterating the mastoid air cell system without interfering with the external meatus, ossicles or tympanic membrane (Fig. 38).

Radical and modified radical mastoidectomy for cholesteatoma involve removal of the posterior meatal wall creating a large cavity accessible for cleaning (Fig. 39).

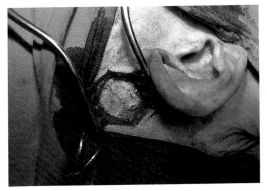

Fig. 37 Harvesting a temporalis fascia graft.

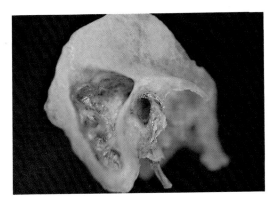

Fig. 38 Cortical mastoidectomy (cadaver dissection).

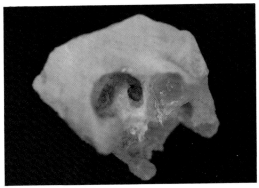

Fig. 39 Radical mastoidectomy (cadaver dissection).

12 / Facial nerve palsy

Disruption of the lower motor neurone facial nerve can occur at any point between its brainstem nucleus and the facial musculature.

Bell's (idiopathic) palsy

Clinical features
Most common palsy with no identifiable cause although a viral or vascular aetiology postulated. Palsy may be partial or complete.

Management
Total recovery occurs in 90% of cases. Treatment with steroids or surgical decompression controversial.

Ramsay Hunt syndrome

Clinical features
Herpes zoster involvement of the facial nerve with herpetic vesicles on the tympanic membrane (Fig. 40), pinna (Fig. 41) or palate. May present with severe otalgia alone. Auditory and trigeminal nerves may be affected.

Management
Recovers fully in about 60% of cases. If given early the antiviral agent acyclovir may enhance recovery. The value of steroids or surgical decompression of the nerve remains unproven.

Temporal bone fracture

Clinical features
Longitudinal fractures (80%) are associated with a facial palsy in 20% of cases, and a conductive deafness. Transverse fractures (20%) are associated with a facial palsy in 50% of cases, and a sensorineural deafness.

Management
Exploration of the nerve may be indicated in cases of immediate, complete paralysis but is likely to be followed by deafness.

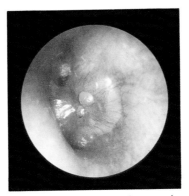

Fig. 40 Herpetic vesicules on the tympanic membrane.

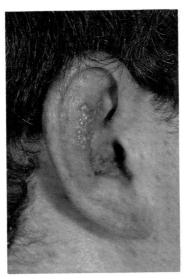

Fig. 41 Herpetic vesicles on the pinna.

13 / Otogenic vertigo

Otogenic vertigo is the creation of a false sensation of movement. Disease affecting the vestibular apparatus may produce rotatory vertigo accompanied by horizontal nystagmus.

Testing **Caloric testing** (Fig. 42). Involves stimulating the vestibular apparatus by irrigating the external meatus with water at varying temperatures; the duration of induced nystagmus is recorded allowing comparison between the two sides.

Positional testing. Vertigo provoked by head movements (positional vertigo) (Fig. 43) may be a feature of inner ear disease, cervical spondylosis or disease affecting central vestibular pathways in the brainstem.

Menière's disease

Aetiology Unknown, may be due to imbalance between production and absorption of inner ear endolymph, or disturbance of inner ear immunity.

Clinical features Episodic rotatory vertigo, tinnitus and sensorineural deafness may be present. Unilateral in early stages.

Management Treat with vestibular sedatives for acute attacks. Surgical treatment may be conservative (endolymphatic sac surgery) or destructive (labyrinthectomy or vestibular nerve section), and is reserved for severe cases.

Sudden unilateral vestibular failure

Aetiology Unknown aetiology. Viral infection, ischaemia and inner ear membrane rupture have been postulated.

Clinical features Presents with sudden onset of vertigo. Recovery takes place by central compensation.

Management Vestibular sedatives are useful in the acute phase.

Other causes of vertigo are syphilis, suppurative labyrinthitis, temporal fractures and ototoxic drugs, particularly aminoglycoside antibiotics.

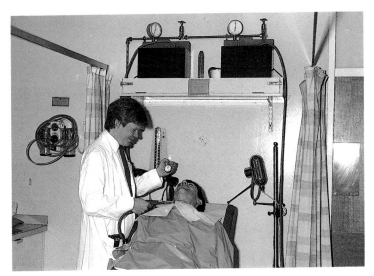

Fig. 42 Caloric testing.

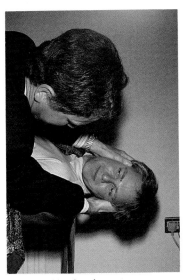

Fig. 43 Positional testing.

14 / Sensorineural hearing loss

Sensorineural hearing loss results from disease in the cochlea or its central neuronal connections. The disease can be congenital (Fig. 44) or acquired.

Congenital

Aetiology **Aplasias**. Partial or complete failure of inner ear development, e.g. Schiebe anomaly.

Abiotrophies. Inner ear anatomically developed but neural pathways degenerate prematurely, e.g. Pendred, Hurler and Alport syndromes.

Intrauterine/perinatal damage. Includes hypoxia, kernicterus, rubella, cytomegalovirus, syphilis, thalidomide.

Acquired

Aetiology
- Presbyacusis: the most common cause.
- Noise-induced hearing loss.
- Menière's disease.
- Acoustic neuroma (Fig. 45).
- Trauma, e.g. head injury, middle ear surgery.
- Sudden (idiopathic) sensorineural hearing loss.
- Drug-induced hearing loss, e.g. gentamicin (Fig. 46).
- Syphilis/yaws.

Management The management of any sensorineural hearing loss involves rehabilitation, once any treatable cause has been excluded. Special schooling may be necessary for the severely deaf child.

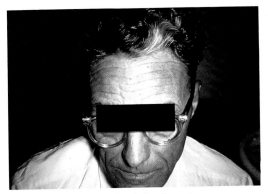

Fig. 44 White forelock in Waardenburg's syndrome.

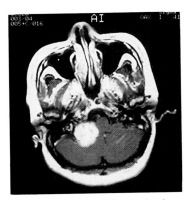

Fig. 45 Posterior fossa MRI scan showing an acoustic neuroma.

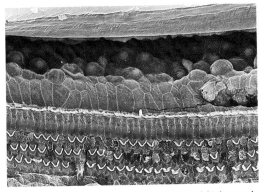

Fig. 46 Scanning electron micrograph of gentamicin-damaged cochlear hair cells.

15 / Rehabilitation of deafness

Early diagnosis of deafness is the key to successful auditory rehabilitation, particularly in children with congenital deafness. With early intensive auditory training most children will develop the ability to communicate orally. Lip reading is an adjunct to oral communication. Manual communication, as in sign language, may be applicable for severely deaf people.

Hearing aids

Hearing aids amplify incoming sound and in some cases modify the frequency response and maximum intensity. The postaural aid (Fig. 47) is most widely used, while the body-worn aid is a bulkier but more powerful alternative. To enable parents to communicate with deaf children the 'phonic aid' (Fig. 48) has been developed in which sound is transmitted electronically over short distances.

Cochlear implants

Direct electrical stimulation of the cochlear portion of the inner ear in response to incoming sound waves has been investigated in the development of cochlear implants. Electrodes are either placed on the surface of the cochlea (extracochlear) or inserted into the lumen of the cochlea (intracochlear) (Fig. 49).

The use of cochlear implantation is established in patients with severe sensorineural deafness (e.g. post-meningitis). It is currently being evaluated in children with congenital deafness.

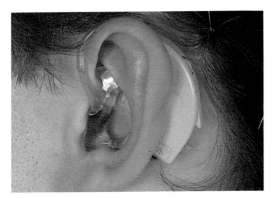

Fig. 47 Postaural hearing aid.

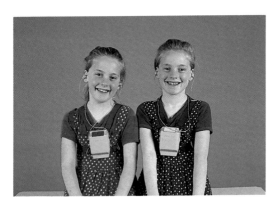

Fig. 48 Phonic aids.

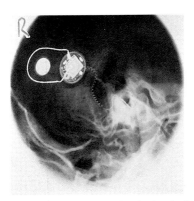

Fig. 49 X-ray showing cochlear implant in situ.

16 / Diseases of the external nose

Rhinophyma

Clinical features
Red nodular masses centred around the nasal tip in association with acne rosacea (Fig. 50), usually seen in elderly men.

Management
If unsightly, treat by dermabrasion or surgical shaving.

Lupus vulgaris

Aetiology
Inoculation of the bacterium *Mycobacterium tuberculosis* possibly through nose–picking.

Clinical features
Red/brown patches or nodules on the nasal or facial skin. Perforation of the cartilaginous nasal septum can occur, with scarring in long–standing cases (Fig. 51).

Management
Treatment is by antituberculous chemotherapy.

Lupus pernio

Clinical features
Skin lesions other than erythema nodosum occur in 20% of patients with sarcoidosis. Lupus pernio (Fig. 52) is common and is frequently associated with bone cysts and chest disease.

Management
Treat the underlying disease.

Malignant tumours

Clinical features
Basal or squamous cell carcinomas (Fig. 53) present as warty or ulcerating lesions, rarely with lymphadenopathy. Melanomas are more rare.

Management
Excision biopsy when possible; radiotherapy for larger tumours not involving bone.

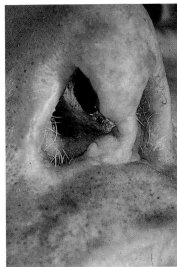

Fig. 50 Rhinophyma.

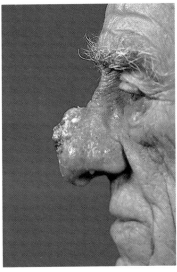

Fig. 51 Lupus vulgaris.

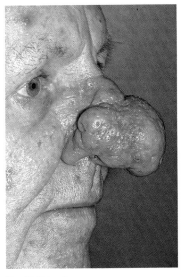

Fig. 52 Lupus pernio.

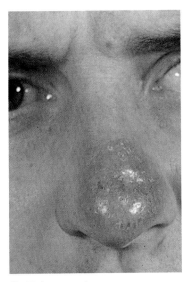

Fig. 53 Squamous carcinoma.

17 / **Epistaxis**

Aetiology Most cases of epistaxis are idiopathic, although bleeding can also result from a number of specific conditions.

- *Local conditions*: include nasal trauma, nasal and paranasal sinus tumours and nasal septal perforations.
- *General conditions*: include systemic bleeding diatheses such as leukaemia, anticoagulant therapy and thrombocytopenia, and systemic vascular disorders. In hereditary haemorrhagic telangiectasia (Rendu-Osler-Weber syndrome, Fig. 54) epistaxis is a prominent feature and usually arises from abnormal vessels on the nasal septum.

Systemic hypertension although not a cause of epistaxis is often associated with an increased severity of bleeding.

Clinical features In most cases of epistaxis bleeding originates from the nasal septum, particularly Little's area just behind the mucocutaneous junction where there is a rich anastomosis of vessels (Kiesselbach's plexus, Fig. 55). Bleeding may occur through the anterior nares or pass backwards via the nasopharynx where it is spat out or swallowed. In severe cases with profuse blood loss hypotension and tachycardia may occur.

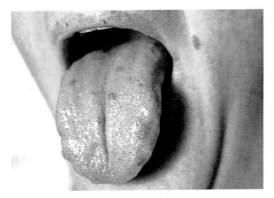

Fig. 54 Rendu-Osler-Weber syndrome.

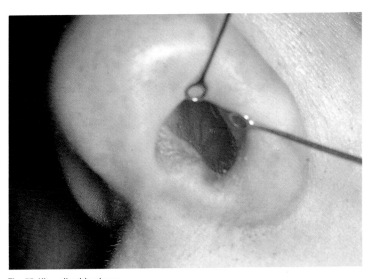

Fig. 55 Kiesselbach's plexus.

Management   Initial measures to stop bleeding consist of exerting
pressure on Little's area by pinching the nose, with
the patient leaning forward and spitting any blood
into a bowl (Fig. 56). If a bleeding vessel is seen it
may be coagulated with chemical or electric cautery
following topical application of local anaesthetic, but
this is rarely successful in the acute stage. Epistaxis
not responding to pressure necessitates nasal packing
either with gauze impregnated with an antiseptic such
as bismuth, iodoform and paraffin paste (BIPP)
(Fig. 57), or with nasal balloons. Patients requiring
nasal packing also require hospitalisation.

In severe cases arterial ligation may be required,
with available arteries being the external carotid via
the neck (Fig. 58), the internal maxillary via the
maxillary antrum and the anterior ethmoidal via an
inner canthal incision.

An alternative to arterial ligation in severe cases is
arterial embolisation performed with angiographic
control by a radiologist. Intravenous resuscitation with
blood or plasma substitute is necessary in cases where
hypotension and tachycardia are present.

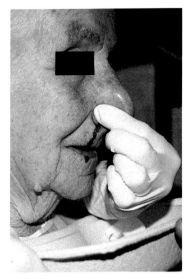

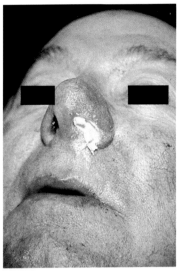

Fig. 56 Pressure and posture during epistaxis.

Fig. 57 Nasal packing.

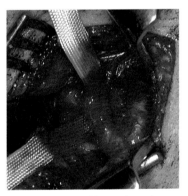

Fig. 58 External carotid artery just prior to ligation.

18 / Diseases of the nasal septum

Deviated nasal septum

Aetiology This occurs following previous nasal trauma or results from asymmetric septal development possibly following birth trauma.

Clinical features Presents as unilateral nasal obstruction (Fig. 59) and less commonly epistaxis. The inferior and middle turbinates on the side opposite the septal deflection often undergo compensatory hypertrophy.

Management If symptoms warrant the septum can be positioned in the midline as in the operations of septoplasty and submucosal resection.

Septal haematoma

A collection of blood beneath the mucoperichondrium and posteriorly the mucoperiosteum of the nasal septum.

Aetiology Usually complicates nasal trauma, either accidental or iatrogenic following septal surgery. Rarely a spontaneous haematoma can occur in a bleeding diathesis.

Clinical features Presents as nasal obstruction with widening of the septum on inspection (Fig. 60).

Management In the acute stage, treat by incision and drainage; however, after 48 hours, organisation of haematoma occurs and evacuation of the clot is difficult. Antibiotics are given to prevent secondary infection.

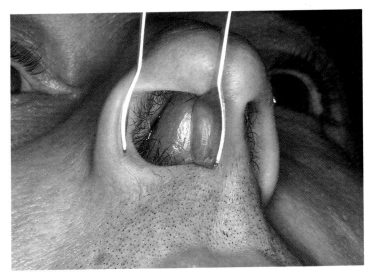

Fig. 59 Deviated nasal septum.

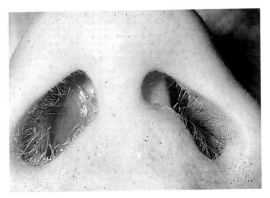

Fig. 60 Septal haematoma.

Septal abscess

Aetiology Septal abscesses usually result from secondary infection of a septal haematoma.

Clinical features Manifests by the development of severe pain, nasal swelling and pyrexia following a septal haematoma. Cartilage necrosis often complicates septal haematoma and abscess with the production of a saddle-nose deformity (Fig. 61).

Management Treatment is by incision and drainage with appropriate antibiotic therapy.

Septal perforation

Aetiology ***Traumatic***: after septal surgery, nose picking, cocaine sniffing and pressure from foreign bodies and nasal polyps.

Infective: due to syphilis and tuberculosis.

Chronic inflammatory. Wegener's granulomatosis is a non-neoplastic upper airways granuloma associated with focal lung and kidney lesions. (Lethal) midline granuloma is thought to be an atypical lymphoma occurring in the midline of the face.

Clinical features Asymptomatic, or nasal crusting and epistaxis are characteristic of septal perforation (Fig. 62).

Management Treatment is by removal of crusts, nasal douches and treatment of underlying systemic conditions.

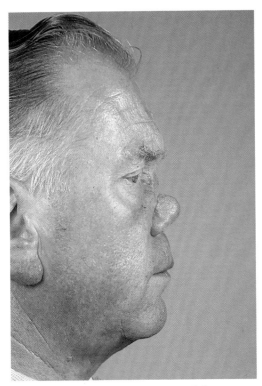

Fig. 61 Saddle-nose deformity following septal abscess.

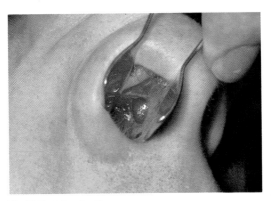

Fig. 62 Septal perforation.

19 / Non-infective rhinitis

Allergic rhinitis

Aetiology Hypersensitivity to inhaled or ingested allergens causes nasal mucosal oedema and exudation. Allergy may be seasonal (e.g. pollens) or perennial (e.g. house dust). Allergies may be demonstrated by skin tests (Fig. 63).

Clinical features Presents as nasal obstruction, sneezing and rhinorrhoea with mucosal oedema on examination (Fig. 64).

Management Treat with steroid nasal spray and oral antihistamines. Avoid any known allergens.

Non-allergic rhinitis

Clinical features Presents as chronic nasal obstruction and rhinorrhoea with no demonstrable allergy.

Management If medical treatment in the form of antihistamines or steroid sprays fail to produce relief, nasal obstruction may be helped by surgical reduction or diathermy of the inferior turbinates.

Long term use of sympathomimetic vasoconstrictor nasal sprays can result in chronic nasal congestion as a rebound effect—rhinitis medicamentosa.

Atrophic rhinitis

Aetiology A disease of unknown aetiology, occurring mainly in developing countries. It can occur following radical turbinectomy operations or radiotherapy to the nasal cavity.

Clinical features Nasal crusting, anosmia and foetor are present. Paradoxically, although the nasal cavity is widely patent, the sensation of nasal obstruction is common.

Management Treatment is by removal of crusts and nasal douches.

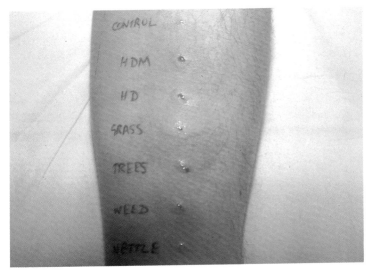

Fig. 63 Positive skin tests in allergic rhinitis.

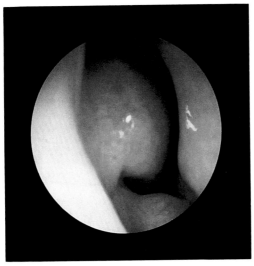

Fig. 64 Inferior turbinate hypertrophy.

20 / Simple nasal polyps

Aetiology Simple nasal polyps are pedunculated areas of oedematous mucosa occurring in the nasal cavity and paranasal sinuses. Their aetiology is unknown although chronic sinus infection and mucosal allergy have been suggested. Most polyps arise from the ethmoid sinuses with the maxillary antrum being a less common source.

Nasal polyps can be associated with asthma and aspirin sensitivity (aspirin triad). In children, nasal polyps may be a manifestation of cystic fibrosis.

Clinical features Presents as progressive nasal obstruction and rhinorrhoea. On inspection of the nasal cavity polyps are seen as pale grey smooth swellings which can fill the nasal cavity (Fig. 65). Most cases are bilateral but in unilateral cases a neoplasm must be excluded by biopsy. An antrochoanal polyp passes from the maxillary sinus via its ostium posteriorly into the nasal cavity to occupy the posterior choana where it can be seen on posterior rhinoscopy (Fig. 66) and its presence confirmed by lateral radiography.

Management **Medical treatment** with topical steroid drops or spray administered correctly can cause considerable diminution in polyp size.

Surgical treatment in the form of intranasal polypectomy (Fig. 67) may have to be repeated as recurrence after polyp removal is common. In severe cases ethmoidectomy may be required.

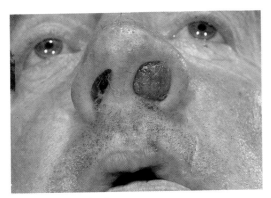

Fig. 65 Simple nasal polyps.

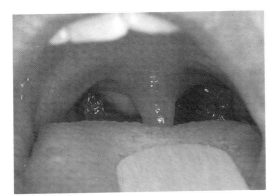

Fig. 66 Antrochoanal polyp behind soft palate.

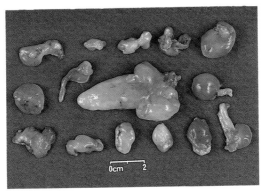

Fig. 67 Operative specimens from one patient.

21 / Acute sinusitis

Aetiology Stasis and acute infection of sinus secretions may result from any pathological or anatomical abnormality obstructing free sinus drainage. The common cold is the most frequent cause. Acute maxillary sinusitis can also result from apical infection of an upper tooth root. The causative organism is usually *Pneumococcus, Streptococcus viridans* or *Haemophilus influenzae.*

Complications Left untreated, acute sinusitis can rarely lead to orbital cellulitis, cavernous sinus thrombosis or frontal lobe abscess formation. Chronic sinusitis is a far more common sequal.

Maxillary sinusitis

Clinical features Most common type overall. Facial or dental pain may occur, as may referred otalgia. Nasal obstruction and purulent rhinorrhoea are also frequent. Local tenderness may be the only physical sign. An occipito-mental X-ray usually shows a fluid level on one or both sides (Fig. 68).

Management Treat with antibiotics and topical nasal decongestants. An antral washout (Fig. 69) through the inferior meatus may be necessary if resolution with antibiotics does not occur, but this form of treatment is decreasing in popularity with the advent of endoscopic management of sinusitis.

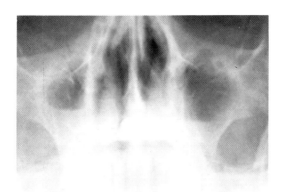

Fig. 68 Bilateral antral fluid levels.

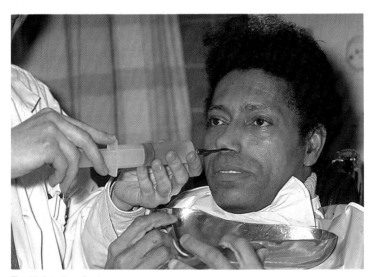

Fig. 69 Antral washout.

Ethmoiditis

Incidence Most common in young children who have poorly developed maxillary sinuses.

Clinical features Usually presents as persistent headache and orbital cellulitis (Fig. 70) following a cold. Untreated, an orbital abscess and blindness may occur.

Management Treatment requires hospital admission. Antibiotics are given and the maxillary sinuses washed out if also infected. Rarely, an external ethmoidectomy may be necessary. A CT scan should be performed if there is any question of an orbital abscess.

Frontal sinusitis

Potentially the most serious acute sinusitis. The long course of the frontonasal duct makes it particularly prone to obstruction by mucosal oedema.

Clinical features Presents as frontal headache after an upper respiratory tract infection. Local tenderness is common, but may be the only sign. An occipito-frontal X-ray usually shows a fluid level or complete opacification in one or both sinuses.

Management Treatment is with antibiotics, but sinus trephine and insertion of drainage tubes (Fig. 71) is undertaken if rapid resolution does not occur.

Sphenoiditis

Clinical features This rare form of sinusitis may present as a deep central, retro-orbital or vertex headache. Diagnosis is confirmed by a lateral X-ray or CT scan (Fig. 72). Sinus drainage may be necessary if there is not a quick response to antibiotic therapy.

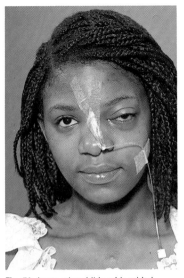

Fig. 70 Acute ethmoiditis with orbital cellulitis.

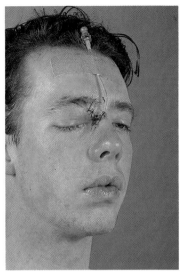

Fig. 71 Surgical drainage of acute frontal sinusitis.

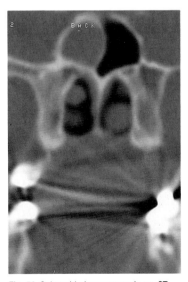

Fig. 72 Sphenoid sinus mucocele on CT scan.

22 / Chronic sinusitis

Frontal sinusitis

Clinical features

Presents as a persistent frontal headache or, if a mucocele develops, a unilateral proptosis (Fig. 73). A pyocele may result from secondary infection of a mucocele. X-rays show an opaque sinus often with hazy, indistinct edges. A CT scan will show a soft tissue mass filling the sinus (Fig. 74).

Management

Treatment is by a fronto-ethmoidectomy, leaving a polythene tube in situ for three months in order to re-establish a good frontonasal duct. Further problems merit frontal sinus obliteration via an osteoplastic flap approach.

Maxillary sinusitis

Aetiology

Disease is commonly bilateral unless there is an underlying septal deviation, unilateral polyp or history of maxillary trauma. A past history of dental treatment may be relevant.

Clinical features

Usually presents with chronic facial pain or upper jaw toothache. Other presentations include a purulent postnasal drip, chronic laryngitis or otitis media. Examination is often normal but paranasal sinus X-rays usually demonstrate antral disease, either in the form of mucosal thickening, a persistent fluid level or total opacification.

Management

Treatment involves the creation of intranasal antrostomies to drain the antra. If symptoms persist a Caldwell-Luc approach can be used to remove the diseased antral mucosa (Fig. 75).

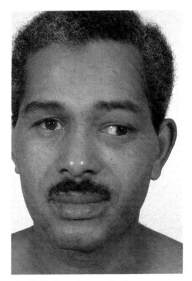

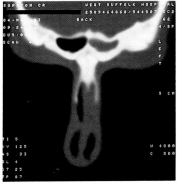

Fig. 73 Unilateral proptosis due to a mucocele.

Fig. 74 Unilateral chronic frontal sinusitis.

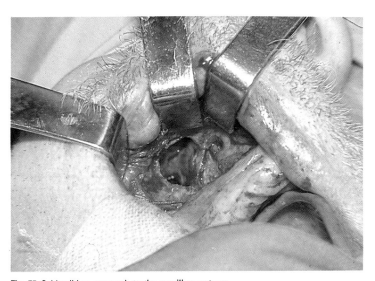

Fig. 75 Caldwell-Luc approach to the maxillary antrum.

23 / Functional endoscopic sinus surgery

The widespread availability of endoscopes and high quality radiology has led to a reappraisal of many of the established methods of treatment for chronic sinusitis. Most sinus infections are rhinogenic, spreading from the nose into the sinuses. Both the frontal and maxillary sinuses are drained and ventilated through the narrow clefts of the anterior ethmoid cells, close to the middle nasal turbinate. It is this small area which is critical in the development of chronic sinusitis.

Diagnostic evaluation

Patients with a history suggestive of chronic sinusitis are evaluated by rigid endoscopy under local anaesthetic. The middle meatus is particularly important (Fig. 76), and is inspected for evidence of polyps, purulent secretion (Fig. 77) or anatomical abnormality which may impede sinus ventilation.

Where endoscopic surgery is necessary a CT scan in the coronal plane is obtained to show the underlying sinus anatomy (Fig. 78), the extent of chronic sinus disease (Fig. 79), and the relationship to adjacent structures such as the orbital contents and anterior cranial fossa.

Endoscopic surgery

When chronic sinusitis persists despite adequate medical treatment patients may undergo endoscopic surgery. These operations remove diseased sinus mucosa and improve ventilation in the middle meatus area. Usually anterior ethmoidectomy is performed, but in more extensive disease access to the posterior ethmoidal and sphenoidal sinuses is possible.

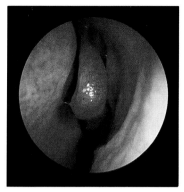

Fig. 76 Normal middle meatus.

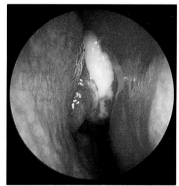

Fig. 77 Pus in the middle meatus.

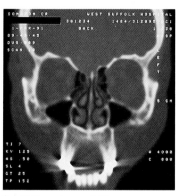

Fig. 78 Normal coronal CT scan.

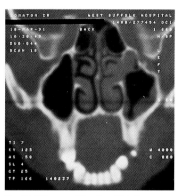

Fig. 79 CT scan with ethmoidal disease.

24 / Adenoids

Lymphoid tissue found at the junction of the roof and posterior wall of the nasopharynx, thought to be involved in the development of humoral immunity as a component of the 'gut associated lymphoid tissue' (GALT). Adenoid tissue is present at birth and during childhood, beginning to atrophy before puberty.

Clinical features

Adenoidal hypertrophy (Fig. 80) disturbs nasopharyngeal airflow and eustachian tube function and can also act as a focus of infection for adjacent sites. Common clinical features are nasal obstruction and discharge, deafness due to middle ear effusion and otalgia due to recurrent otitis media. Gross adenoidal enlargement often associated with tonsillar hypertrophy can cause the sleep apnoea syndrome in which apnoeic episodes during sleep are associated with daytime somnolence and in severe cases pulmonary hypertension and cor pulmonale. Clinical suspicion of enlarged adenoids can be confirmed by lateral radiography (Fig. 81).

Management

Surgical removal (adenoidectomy) can be undertaken if enlarged adenoids are causing sleep apnoea, nasal obstruction or are a contributing factor to persistent middle effusions or recurrent otitis media.

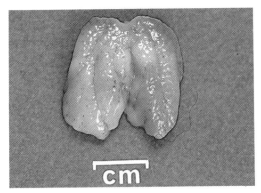

Fig. 80 Operative specimen of adenoids.

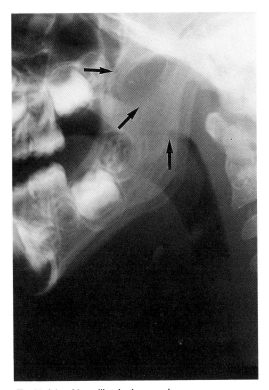

Fig. 81 Adenoid swelling·in the nasopharynx.

25 / Facial fractures

Nasal fractures

Clinical features

This common fracture can produce an external deformity (Fig. 82), which may be palpable, and internal disruption, e.g. septal haematoma or septal deviation. Ethmoid involvement may produce CSF rhinorrhoea.

Management

Reduce any external bony deviation under general or local anaesthesia. A septal deviation may require a submucosal resection at a later date.

Zygomatic (malar) fractures

Clinical features

Usually tripartite (Fig. 83), the cheek contour is flattened and trismus is common. Orbital movements may be limited if the orbital floor is involved.

Management

Elevation of the zygoma (via a Gillies approach) may need to be supplemented by internal wiring and antral packing, through a Caldwell-Luc approach.

Maxillary (Le Fort) fractures

There are three types of maxillary or Le Fort fracture (Fig. 84):
• Type I
• Type II
• Type III

Clinical features

Airways obstruction by the mobile bone fragment is a serious threat. Malocclusion is common.

Management

Treatment involves fixing the mobile portion using arch bars and, frequently, bilateral suspension wiring from the frontal or parietal bones.

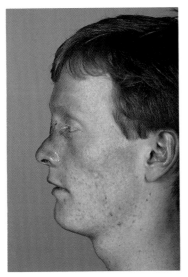

Fig. 82 Fractured nasal bones.

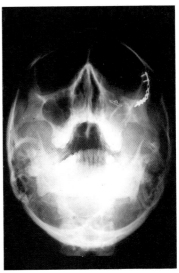

Fig. 83 Zygomatic fracture after open reduction.

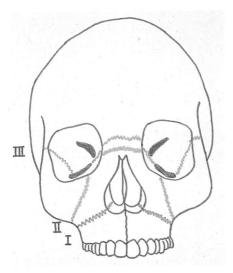

Fig. 84 Types of Le Fort maxillary fractures.

26 / Tumours of the nasopharynx

Angiofibroma

Incidence　A benign vascular tumour occurring in males under the age of 25 years.

Clinical features　Nasal obstruction, epistaxis and deafness due to middle ear effusion are common characteristics.

Management　Treatment is by surgical excision, facilitated by preoperative CT scanning (Fig. 85), arteriography and embolisation (Fig. 86).

Malignant tumours

Incidence　Common in South East Asia where they account for 20% of all malignant tumours.

Clinical features　Presents as nasal obstruction, epistaxis and deafness. Metastasis to cervical nodes may occur prior to local symptoms becoming apparent (Fig. 87). Cranial nerve palsies occur in advanced cases.

Pathology　Most are squamous carcinomas, although anaplastic carcinomas and lymphomas also occur.

Management　Radiotherapy, with surgery used only for cervical nodes not responding to irradiation.

Chordoma

A very rare locally invasive neoplasm arising from remnants of the fetal notochord found in the skull base. Presents with neurological, nasal and ophthalmic symptoms.

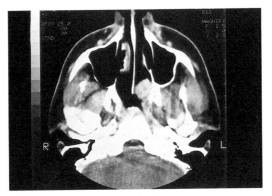

Fig. 85 CT scan showing an angiofibroma.

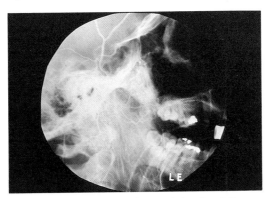

Fig. 86 Arteriogram demonstrating vascularity of angiofibroma.

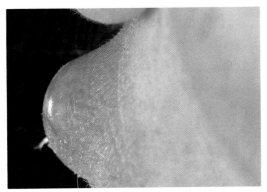

Fig. 87 Malignant neck nodes secondary to nasopharyngeal carcinoma.

27 / Paranasal sinus tumours

Pathology **Benign tumours**. These include papillomas, adenomas, osteomas and angiomas. The inverting papilloma may undergo malignant change.

Malignant tumours. 50% of malignant tumours are found in the maxillary sinus. Squamous cell carcinoma is the most common type. Others include adenocarcinoma, adenoid cystic carcinoma, melanoma and sarcoma.

Clinical features Benign tumours frequently present as a unilateral nasal polyp. Malignant tumours spread medially to produce nasal obstruction or epistaxis, posteriorly to give eustachian tube obstruction and cranial nerve palsies, inferiorly to disrupt the teeth (Fig. 88) or superiorly to give proptosis or epiphora. Lateral spread produces swelling of the cheek.

Management Prior to treatment planning, histological diagnosis and radiological assessment of the extent of the tumour using CT scanning and sinus tomography are necessary (Fig. 89). Benign tumours are treated by local excision, e.g. by a Caldwell-Luc or lateral rhinotomy approach. Malignant tumours have a poor prognosis due to their late presentation and extensive spread. When curative treatment is possible a combination of radical surgery (maxillectomy) and radiotherapy is usually used. The resulting defect is filled with a dental plate and obturator (Fig. 90).

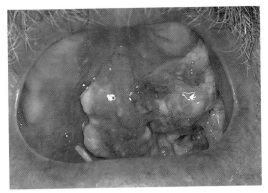

Fig. 88 Antral carcinoma involving hard palate.

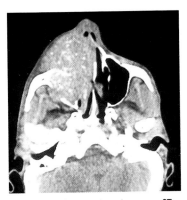

Fig. 89 Extensive antral carcinoma on CT scan.

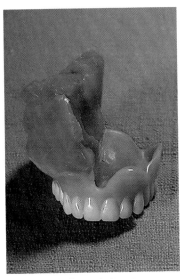

Fig. 90 Dental plate and obturator.

28 / Nasal airway obstruction in children

Nasal obstruction in children is usually noted by parents particularly when accompanied by rhinorrhoea and snoring. Adenoid hypertrophy is the commonest cause of paediatric nasal obstruction; however, the following conditions should also be borne in mind.

Posterior choanal atresia

Aetiology

A congenital condition caused by persistence of the embryonic bucconasal membrane. The obstruction is at the posterior end of the nose near the edge of the hard palate.

Clinical features

In bilateral cases there is respiratory difficulty at birth aggravated by feeding and necessitating the use of an oral airway. Unilateral cases present later with unilateral nasal obstruction and rhinorrhoea. Diagnosis is made by the inability to pass a rubber catheter through the nose into the pharynx and is confirmed by CT scanning (Fig. 91).

Management

Surgical division of the atretic plate by transnasal or transpalatal route is required.

Nasal foreign body

A common occurrence in children, e.g. with beads, pieces of sponge or paper (Fig. 92).

Clinical features

Typically presents with unilateral foul blood-stained rhinorrhoea, nasal vestibulitis and foetor.

Management

A general anaesthetic is occasionally required for removal in an uncooperative child.

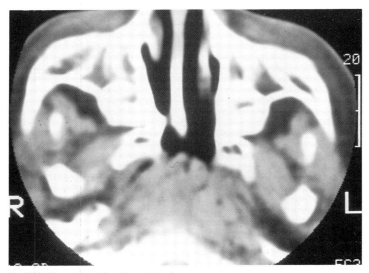

Fig. 91 Unilateral posterior choanal atresia.

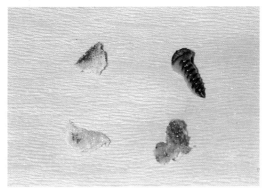

Fig. 92 Foreign bodies removed from a child's nose.

29 / Laryngeal obstruction in children

Clinical features The hallmark of laryngeal obstruction is stridor. Inspiratory stridor indicates glottic or supraglottic obstruction, expiratory stridor bronchial obstruction and two-way stridor subglottic obstruction. If stridor is accompanied by cyanosis, tachycardia and intercostal and sternal recession (Fig. 93) urgent measures are needed to save life. In less severe cases a hoarse voice, feeding problems and recurrent chest infections may occur.

Congenital laryngeal obstruction

Aetiology Congenital anomalies include laryngeal cysts, webs, stenosis, vascular rings and vocal cord paralysis. Laryngomalacia is a condition caused by abnormal flaccidity of the larynx allowing the supraglottic structures to be drawn into the airway on inspiration; the condition resolves with age.

Management All cases of congenital stridor should undergo direct laryngoscopy.

Acquired laryngeal obstruction

Aetiology ***Acute epiglottitis***: due to *Haemophilus infuenzae*. It causes rapidly progressive airway obstruction (Fig. 94).

Acute laryngotracheobronchitis (croup): due to para-influenzae virus or respiratory syncitial virus. It produces oedema, exudates and crusting of the larynx, trachea and bronchi.

Subglottic stenosis: may follow infant tracheostomy or prolonged endotracheal intubation.

Management ***Acute epiglottitis***: treatment is with intravenous chloramphenicol. Endotracheal intubation or an emergency tracheostomy may be necessary.

Acute laryngotracheobronchitis: endotracheal intubation is rarely required.

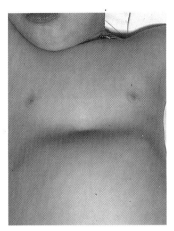

Fig. 93 Sternal recession in a child with upper airways obstruction.

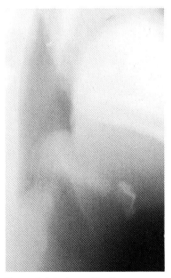

Fig. 94 Epiglottic swelling in acute epiglottitis.

30 / Acute tonsillitis

Incidence A very common disease particularly affecting children between the ages of 4 and 10 years.

Aetiology Over 50% of the cases are due to a B haemolytic streptococcus, the majority of the others being of viral, staphylococcal or pneumococcal origin.

Clinical features Sore throat, dysphagia, pain on swallowing and otalgia are associated with pyrexia and general malaise. The pharyngeal mucosa appears red and the tonsils are often enlarged and covered by discrete microabscesses or a confluent exudate (Fig. 95). The tonsils often remain chronically enlarged and inflamed (Fig. 96). Lymphadenopathy is frequent, the jugulo-digastric nodes being most commonly involved. A full blood count reveals a leucocytosis but a bacteriology swab does not always grow the pathogen concerned.

Differential diagnosis ***Infectious mononucleosis***. It may be impossible to distinguish between the two without a Paul-Bunnell test and a differential white cell count (the latter shows atypical monocytes and a lymphocytosis).

Blood dyscrasias. Any white cell abnormality giving an impaired immune status may present as a severe pharyngitis, e.g. acute leukaemia.

Diphtheria. Rarely seen but should always be borne in mind when there is a membranous exudate over the tonsils or when severe airways obstruction is evident.

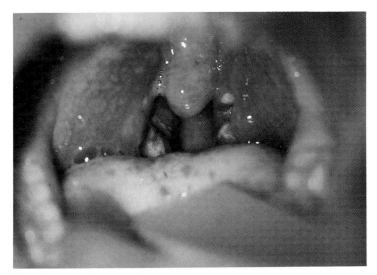

Fig. 95 Acute exudative tonsillitis.

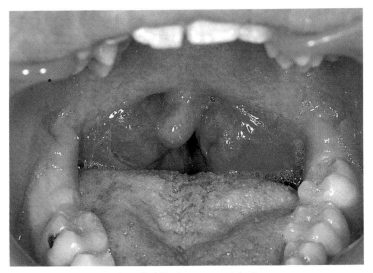

Fig. 96 Chronically enlarged tonsils following recurrent infection.

Management   Bed rest, antibiotics and adequate hydration.
Penicillin is given (orally or intravenously) unless
organism sensitivities or allergy dictate otherwise.
In severe cases with grossly enlarged tonsils a
tracheostomy may be necessary for airways
obstruction.

Recurrent episodes over a prolonged period of time
are best managed by tonsillectomy (Fig. 97).
Following surgery the tonsillar fossae heal over a
period of 7–10 days during which time they are
covered by a slough (Fig. 98) which may mimic an
ulcerative pharyngitis. Infection and secondary
haemorrhage from the fossae can occur during this
period.

Complications
- *Chronic tonsillitis.*
- *Peritonsillar abscess (Quinsy)* (Fig. 99)—
  hospitalisation, antibiotics and intraoral incision
  and drainage are required.
- *Parapharyngeal abscess*—requires surgical drainage
  through an external neck incision.
- *Acute otitis media.*
- *Post-streptococcal rheumatic fever/Glomerulonephritis*—
  now rare.

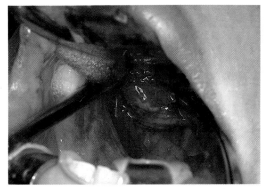

Fig. 97 Dissection tonsillectomy: snaring the lower pole.

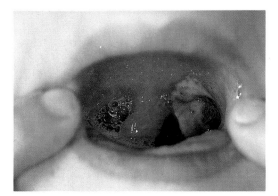

Fig. 98 Post-tonsillectomy slough overlying tonsillar fossae.

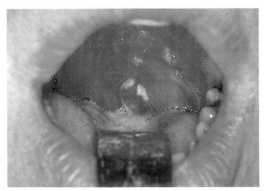

Fig. 99 Left-sided quinsy.

31 / Neck space infections

Acute retropharyngeal abscess

Lymphadenitis of the retropharyngeal nodes following an upper respiratory tract infection in children.

Clinical features
Presents with sore throat, pyrexia and swelling of the posterior pharyngeal wall. Lateral X-ray shows retropharyngeal swelling (Fig. 100).

Management
The abscess should be drained via the mouth with precautions taken to avoid inhalation of pus.

Chronic retropharyngeal abscess

Occurs in adults in association with tuberculous cervical spine disease.

Clinical features
Swelling is seen in the midline of the pharynx and X-rays show vertebral disease.

Management
Treatment is with antituberculous chemotherapy.

Parapharyngeal abscess

The tissue space lateral to the pharynx may become infected by spread of organisms from the tonsils or lower third molar teeth.

Clinical features
Presents with sore throat and trismus. The tonsil is pushed medially and there is neck swelling (Fig. 101).

Management
Treatment is by incision and drainage via the neck followed by appropriate antibiotic therapy.

Ludwig's angina

Clinical features
Cellulitis of the submandibular space secondary to dental disease or tonsillitis presents with swelling of the submental region (Fig. 102) and floor of mouth.

Management
Treat with high dose antibiotics.

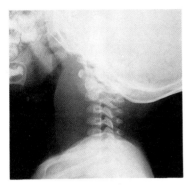

Fig. 100 Retropharyngeal abscess.

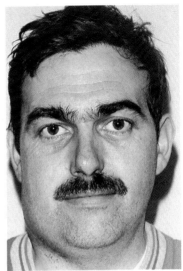

Fig. 101 Parapharyngeal abscess.

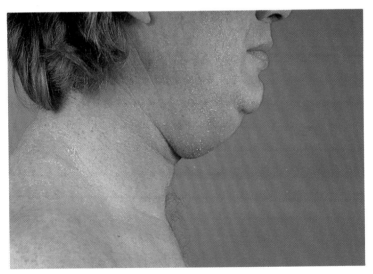

Fig. 102 Ludwig's angina.

32 / Benign conditions of the tongue

Lingual thyroid

Aetiology   Tissue originating from the site of the foramen caecum invaginates and migrates down into the lower neck to form the thyroid gland. Thyroid tissue may be found at any point along this path of descent, e.g. lingual thyroid (Fig. 103) or thyroglossal cyst.

Clinical features   Usually presents as dysphagia. Haemorrhage and airway obstruction rarely occur.

Management   Once functioning thyroid tissue has been demonstrated elsewhere in the neck, the lump may be removed if it is causing significant symptoms.

Black hairy tongue

Aetiology   Caused by overgrowth and elongation of the filiform papillae of the anterior tongue in association with their black or brown discolouration (Fig. 104).

Clinical features   Asymptomatic, but for its appearance.

Management   Treatment is by mechanical brushing or scraping of the dorsum of the tongue.

Geographic tongue

Incidence   Affects 1% of the population.

Clinical features   Irregularly shaped areas of depapillation occur over the dorsum of the tongue (Fig. 105). The patches vary in size and distribution over a period of days.

Management   No treatment is required.

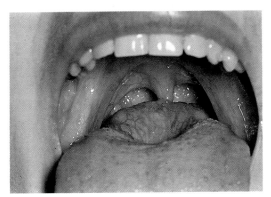

Fig. 103 Lingual thyroid.

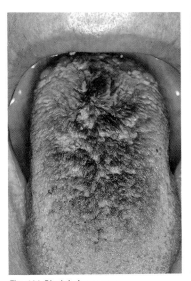

Fig. 104 Black hairy tongue.

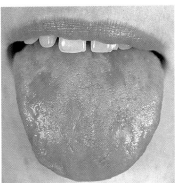

Fig. 105 Geographic tongue.

33 / Leucoplakia and tongue carcinoma

Leucoplakia

A white patch which cannot be wiped away and for which no other diagnosis is apparent (Fig. 106). Risk factors in the development of oral cavity or tongue leucoplakia include alcohol, smoking, spice and betelnut chewing, syphilis and dental trauma. About 5% of cases become malignant. Exclusion of an associated carcinoma is essential.

Tongue carcinoma

Almost all tongue carcinomas are squamous in origin. There need not be any pre-existing leucoplakia.

Clinical features
May present as an exophytic or infiltrative lump on the tongue (Fig. 107). Pain and dysphagia are common. Referred otalgia (via lingual and glossopharyngeal nerves) may also occur. At presentation most tumours are greater than 2 cm diameter and 50% have palpably involved lymph nodes.

Management
Small lesions. Radiotherapy, using external beam or interstitial implant techniques (Fig. 108), or surgery, in the form of a partial or hemi-glossectomy (Fig. 109) are equally effective.

Large lesions. Treatment is with radiotherapy or surgery alone or a planned combination of the two. Both modalities produce quite severe functional disability in the oral cavity, especially regarding speech and swallowing.

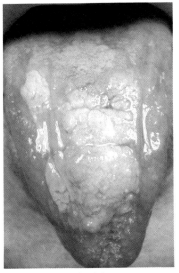

Fig. 106 Leukoplakia of the tongue.

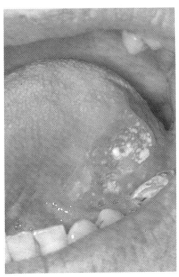

Fig. 107 Ulcerative tongue carcinoma.

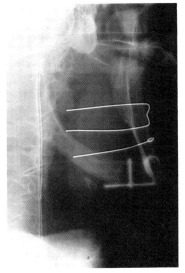

Fig. 108 Interstitial implant in the tongue.

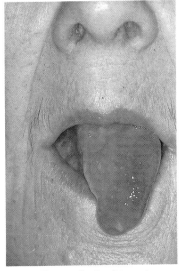

Fig. 109 Tongue after hemiglossectomy.

34 / Tumours of the tonsil

Benign cysts

Clinical features
Mucous retention cysts, tonsilloliths or cysts of inspissated epithelial debris may occur. They are smooth and localised to one portion of the tonsil (Fig. 110).

Management
Symptomatic cysts may be helped by tonsillectomy.

Lymphoma

Clinical features
Unilateral tonsillar swelling with an intact overlying mucosa (Fig. 111) may cause dysphagia and is suspicious of a lymphoma. The tonsil feels rubbery. Excision biopsy confirms the diagnosis.

Management
After staging the disease, treatment involves radiotherapy for localised disease, with chemotherapy being added in more advanced cases.

Carcinoma

Clinical features
Squamous carcinoma of the tonsil presents as otalgia, sore throat or dysphagia in heavy drinkers and smokers. More than 50% of cases have involved neck nodes ipsilaterally: this may be the mode of presentation. The tonsil is hard and ulcerated (Fig. 112).

Management
After full endoscopy and biopsy small primaries without nodes are best treated by radiotherapy. Surgery (which involves a block dissection of neck, partial mandibulectomy and excision of the primary) is reserved for radiation failures and large primaries.

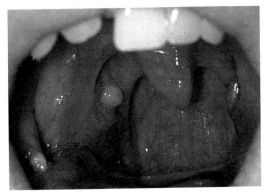

Fig. 110 Tonsil retention cyst.

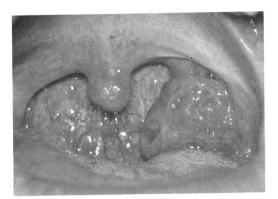

Fig. 111 Tonsil lymphoma.

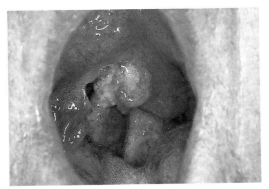

Fig. 112 Carcinoma of the right tonsil.

35 / Diseases of the palate

Torus palatinus

Clinical features   Presents as a unilobular or multilobular bony protruberance in the midline of the hard palate (Fig. 113). The aetiology is unknown.

Management   The torus can be reduced by drilling if a denture needs to be worn or if the swelling interferes with eating.

Palatal tumours

Although these are usually due to inferior extension of a maxillary sinus tumour, benign or malignant neoplasms can arise from the palate itself (Fig. 114).

Clinical features   Presents with loose teeth, ill-fitting dentures and facial swelling. The most common types are the pleomorphic adenoma, adenoid cystic carcinoma and squamous carcinoma.

Management   Treatment is by surgical excision and/or radiotherapy, depending on the histological diagnosis.

Clefts of the palate and lip

Two of the most common congenital anomalies.

Clinical features   Clefts of the lip and palate can occur in isolation (Fig. 115) but they often occur together. Initial difficulties may be encountered with feeding, with abnormal facial development later. Palatal clefts are often associated with middle ear effusions owing to eustachian tube dysfunction.

Management   Plastic surgical repair of clefts with long-term orthodontic care and screening for middle ear effusions.

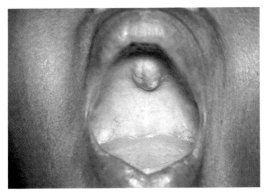

Fig. 113 Torus palatinus.

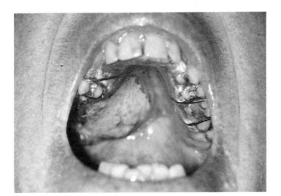

Fig. 114 Pleomorphic adenoma of the hard palate.

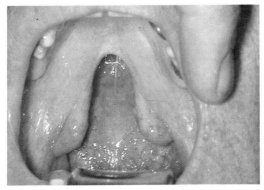

Fig. 115 Untreated cleft palate in an adult.

36 / Chronic laryngitis

Chronic non-specific laryngitis

Aetiology Common. Usually associated with vocal abuse, smoking or sepsis elsewhere in the respiratory tract, e.g. chronic sinusitis.

Clinical features Hoarseness may be accompanied by sore throat. Indirect laryngoscopy may distinguish localised forms, e.g. singer's nodules (Fig. 116), Reinke's oedema (Fig. 117) or laryngeal polyps from the generalised forms, e.g. chronic hypertrophic laryngitis (Fig. 118).

Management Treatment involves the removal of any precipitating factors and speech therapy is important. Localised polyps or nodules may merit endoscopic removal.

Chronic specific laryngitis

Rare. Most of the granulomatous diseases can involve the larynx, e.g. tuberculosis, syphilis, sarcoidosis, scleroma or Wegener's granulomatosis.

Management The lesions may mimic a carcinoma and a direct laryngoscopy and biopsy is mandatory. Treatment is that of the underlying systemic condition.

Leucoplakia

Usually affects the true cords (Fig. 119). The aetiology is as for chronic non-specific laryngitis. Microscopically, the findings of hyperkeratosis and dysplasia are common, although in situ or invasive carcinoma can only be excluded by an adequate biopsy.

Management Endoscopy should be undertaken in all cases. Leucoplakia should be regarded as having the potential to undergo malignant change.

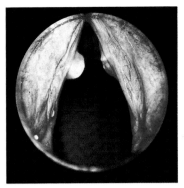

Fig. 116 Singer's nodules.

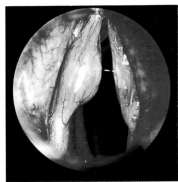

Fig. 117 Unilateral Reinke's oedema.

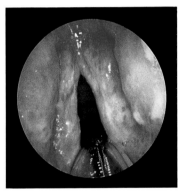

Fig. 118 Chronic hypertrophic laryngitis.

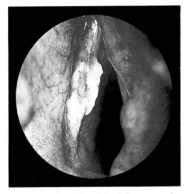

Fig. 119 Leukoplakia of the left true vocal cord.

37 / Laryngeal tumours

Papilloma

Aetiology Localised infection with the human papillomavirus (HPV).

Clinical features **In the child** (juvenile form): multiple lesions which may spread to the trachea and bronchi. Cases may regress at puberty.

In the adult: less common and usually a single lesion.

Both forms present with hoarseness or airway obstruction.

Management Endoscopic removal (Fig. 120) using either suction diathermy or a CO_2 laser. Surgical seeding of lesions within the larynx or trachea is common, and removal may be necessary for frequent recurrence.

Carcinoma

Aetiology Associated with cigarette smoking and high alcohol intake, although the latter is more important in causing piriform fossa carcinoma.

Clinical features Usually presents as persistent hoarseness. Dysphagia, chronic cough, stridor and referred otalgia may also occur. Occasionally a supraglottic tumour may present with metastatic neck nodes. The tumour may be evident on indirect laryngoscopy but endoscopic assessment (Fig. 121) and biopsy is mandatory before deciding on the appropriate treatment. A second primary (1%) in the upper aerodigestive tract should be searched for at this time. Fine needle aspiration cytology of any suspicious neck mass should also be undertaken. A CT scan will show any spread outside the larynx, or involvement of laryngeal cartilages.

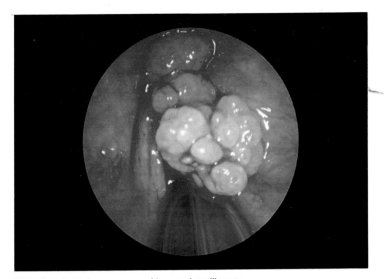

Fig. 120 Endoscopic appearance of laryngeal papillomata.

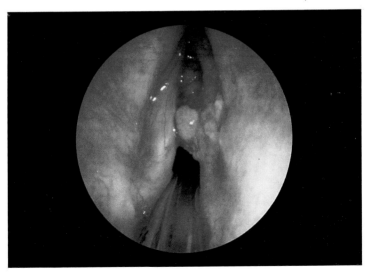

Fig. 121 Early right vocal cord carcinoma.

Management Small (T_1 and T_2) carcinomas are best treated with primary radiotherapy, laryngectomy being reserved for post-radiation recurrences, larger (T_3 and T_4) lesions (Fig. 122) and primary tumours associated with neck nodes greater than 2 cm in diameter.

Voice rehabilitation

Following total laryngectomy the patient may be able to speak again by:
*   learning oesophageal speech (swallowed air is voluntarily regurgitated through the pharynx);
*   using an artificial larynx (Fig. 124) which transmits vibrations into the pharynx and oral cavity while the patient articulates;
*   surgical provision of a tracheo-oesophageal fistula which is fitted with a button or valve (Fig. 123). The button has a one-way flutter valve which allows airflow from the trachea into the pharynx when the tracheostome is occluded. In selected patients this enables the development of good voice.

Results Patients require close follow-up. Recurrences can develop in the larynx, pharynx, stoma or neck. Further surgery or radiotherapy may be indicated. The expected 5-year survival for a T_1 laryngeal cancer is about 95%. This falls to about 50% for T_4 disease.

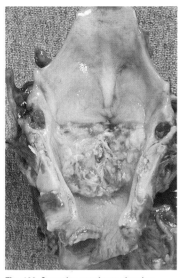

Fig. 122 Operative specimen showing extensive laryngeal carcinoma.

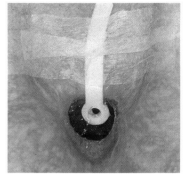

Fig. 123 Blom-Singer valve in situ.

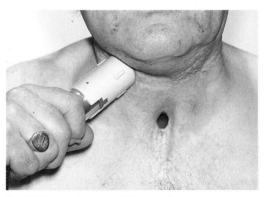

Fig. 124 Patient using an 'artificial larynx'.

38 / Upper aerodigestive tract foreign bodies

Oropharynx

Fish bones may become lodged in the tonsil or tongue base.

Clinical features
The patient complains of pain on swallowing and points to the suprahyoid region on that side. The bone may only be obvious on palpation: X-rays in this area are unhelpful.

Management
Removal under direct vision: occasionally a general anaesthetic is needed.

Hypopharynx/oesophagus

A meat or fish bone or food bolus usually gets lodged at one of four sites:
• one piriform fossa
• the postcricoid region (15 cm from the upper incisor)
• the level of the aortic arch (at 25 cm)
• at the oesophago-gastric junction (40 cm).

Clinical features
Dysphagia may be total, the patient spitting out saliva and pointing to the suprasternal or retrosternal region. A soft tissue lateral X-ray of the neck may delineate a bone (Fig. 125).

Management
Endoscopic removal should be undertaken as soon as possible, to avoid airway oedema, soft tissue infection or oesophageal perforation.

Bronchus

Often a peanut in a young child.

Clinical features
After an initial coughing fit there is often a latent period before symptoms develop. Respiratory distress then becomes obvious. The chest X-ray may show collapse of the lung distally, if the obstruction is complete, or emphysema of the involved side if the obstruction acts as a one-way valve (Fig. 126).

Management
Bronchoscopic removal is mandatory.

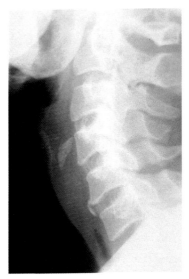

Fig. 125 Chicken bone in hypopharynx.

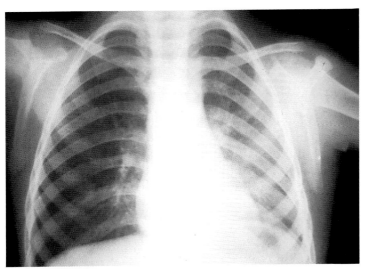

Fig. 126 Peanut in right main bronchus, demonstrating ipsilateral emphysema.

39 / Congenital neck masses

Thyroglossal cyst

Most common midline neck cyst (Fig. 127) usually presenting in childhood.

Clinical features — Painless, unless infected, and moves on protrusion of tongue. Sinus formation may follow previous infection or incomplete excision.

Management — If a thyroid scan shows functioning tissue elsewhere then excise with central portion of hyoid bone and tract up to foramen caecum (Sistrunk's operation).

Branchial cyst and fistula

Aetiology — Represent branchial apparatus remnants. The fistula results from persistence of the second pouch and cervical sinus.

Clinical features — Cysts usually lie deep to the anterior border of sternomastoid, presenting with a painless neck swelling or mimicking a parapharyngeal abscess if infection occurs. A complete branchial fistula has its internal opening in the region of the tonsil and an external opening anterior to sternomastoid. Diagnosis can be confirmed by needle aspiration of cyst contents.

Management — Excision, with any fistulous tract.

Cystic hygroma

A variety of lymphangioma.

Clinical features — A soft, transilluminable mass usually presenting in the parotid region in the first year of life (Fig. 128).

Management — Excision, which may have to be incomplete due to the diffuse infiltration of soft tissues by the tumour.

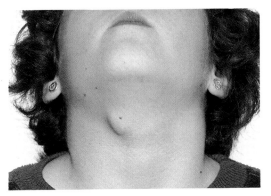

Fig. 127 Thyroglossal cyst.

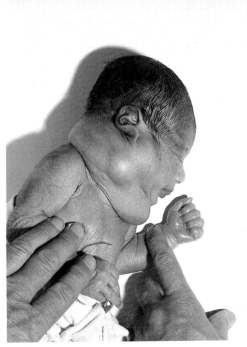

Fig. 128 Cystic hygroma of the right parotid gland.

40 / Tracheostomy

A tracheostomy is an artificial opening made into the trachea. It may be created after the larynx has been removed, when it is permanent, or when the larynx is still in place, when it is usually temporary (Fig. 129).

Indications
- *Total laryngectomy.*
- *Airway protection*, e.g. after major head and neck surgery, neurological disease involving larynx.
- *Airway obstruction*, e.g. epiglottitis, bilateral recurrent laryngeal nerve palsy, tumour.
- *Respiratory insufficiency* (when endotracheal intubation required for longer than 72 hours), e.g. severe chest wall injury, Guillain-Barré syndrome.

Surgical technique
- Incision. Horizontal, midway between the cricoid cartilage and suprasternal notch.
- Vertical incision and separation of strap muscles.
- Transfixion and separation of thyroid isthmus.
- Creation of an opening into the trachea. In adults a window is cut out (Fig. 130). A vertical slit incision is used in children. A trap-door flap should not be used.
- Insertion of tracheostomy tube. A correctly sized cuffed synthetic tube is used for the first 24 hours, following which a silver tube may be used, e.g. Negus-type tracheostomy tube (Fig. 131).

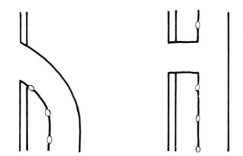

Fig. 129 Types of tracheostomy.

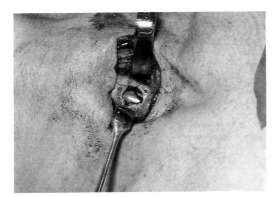

Fig. 130 Window cut in anterior tracheal wall.

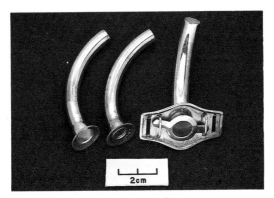

Fig. 131 Silver Negus tracheostomy tubes.

Complications **Immediate**. Pneumothorax, haemorrhage, surgical emphysema and tube displacement can all occur.

Early. Wound infection, dysphagia and tube obstruction are all common. Tracheal erosion with innominate artery rupture, perichondritis and apnoea in hypercapnoeic bronchitics are rare.

Late. Tracheal stenosis may result from prolonged or over inflation of the cuffed tube. Decannulation may be difficult in children. Surgical closure of a persistent tracheocutaneous fistula is rarely required after decannulation.

Stomal stenosis

Aetiology Following laryngectomy the lower end of the trachea is brought out through the neck skin. Local wound infection, radiotherapy, and keloid formation all predispose to the later development of a stomal stenosis (Fig. 132). The other cause of stomal stenosis is recurrence of tumour (Fig. 133).

Management Management of benign stomal stenosis is either by the permanent wearing of a stoma button or laryngectomy tube or by surgical revision of the stoma.

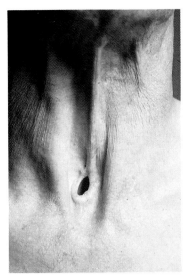

Fig. 132 Stomal stenosis due to scar tissue.

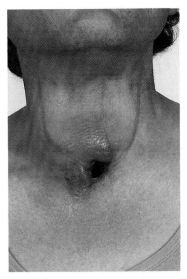

Fig. 133 Post-laryngectomy stomal recurrence.

41 / Diverticulae of the larynx and pharynx

Pharyngeal pouch

Aetiology   A pharyngeal pouch develops from a herniation of pharyngeal mucosa through Killian's dehiscence.

Clinical features   Dysphagia and regurgitation of food occur. Large pouches may cause aspiration pneumonia. Pooling of saliva in the hypopharynx may be noted on indirect laryngoscopy. Barium swallow confirms the diagnosis (Fig. 134).

Management   Following an endoscopy to exclude an associated carcinoma the pouch may be excised, via an external approach, or the wall between the pouch and oesophagus divided endoscopically using Dohlman's procedure (Fig. 135).

Laryngocele

Aetiology   Distension of the laryngeal saccule can produce an internal or an external laryngocele (Fig. 136).

Clinical features   Hoarseness or dysphagia may occur. External laryngoceles may produce a swelling in the neck accentuated by performing Valsalva's manoeuvre. Laryngeal tomograms taken during this manoeuvre will demonstrate the laryngocele (Fig. 137).

Management   Following endoscopy to exclude an associated carcinoma, an internal laryngocele can be 'uncapped' whilst an external laryngocele is excised through the neck.

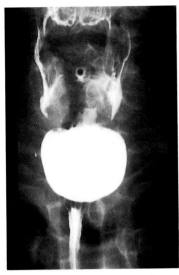

Fig. 134 Barium swallow demonstrating a pharyngeal pouch.

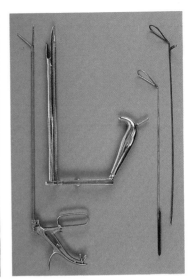

Fig. 135 Dohlman's apparatus.

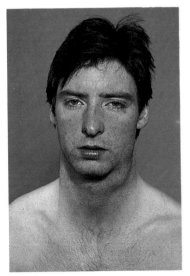

Fig. 136 Patient with an external laryngocele.

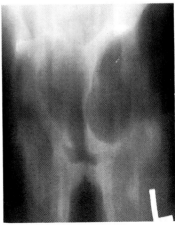

Fig. 137 Tomogram outlining air-filled laryngocele.

42 / Parotid gland swellings

Mumps

Clinical features
Usually seen in children, this is the most common cause of bilateral parotid gland swelling (Fig. 138). The glands are painful and tender.

Management
Treatment is supportive, the adenopathy subsiding over a period of several days.

Acute parotid abscess

Usually seen in association with poor oral hygiene, with or without dental caries.

Clinical features
The gland becomes acutely tender with obvious inflammation of the soft tissues (Fig. 139). A stone may be palpable in the duct or evident on plain X-ray.

Management
Treatment with antibiotics should be followed by drainage via a parotidectomy approach if the swelling becomes fluctuant.

Parotid gland tumours

Types
Benign: e.g. pleomorphic adenoma (Fig. 140), Warthin's tumour.

Malignant: e.g. adenoid cystic, squamous cell or adenocarcinoma, lymphoma.

Clinical features
Usually painless, the speed of growth reflects the likelihood of malignancy. A facial palsy indicates a malignant tumour. Fine needle aspiration of the mass may facilitate preoperative diagnosis.

Management
Superficial parotidectomy should be undertaken when indicated. Malignant tumours may require a total parotidectomy with sacrifice of the facial nerve.

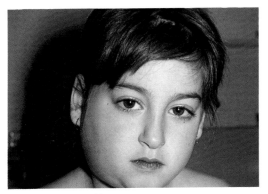

Fig. 138 Mumps parotitis.

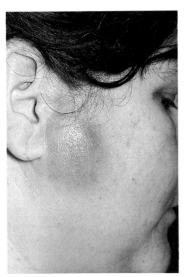

Fig. 139 Acute parotid abscess.

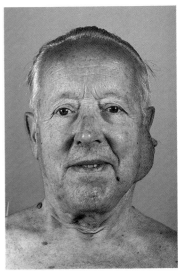

Fig. 140 Pleomorphic adenoma of the parotid gland.

43 / Diseases of the submandibular gland

The superficial portion of the gland lies on the mylohyoid muscle; the deep portion extends around posterior edge of muscle into floor of mouth.
Wharton's duct leaves deep part of gland and runs forward to open into the anterior floor of mouth, just lateral to the midline.

Swelling of the gland may be due to inflammation of tumour (Fig. 141).

Inflammatory disease

Clinical features A tense, tender swelling usually results from a stone in the duct. This may be palpable bi-manually or evident on X-ray (Fig. 142). There are several lymph nodes in the submandibular triangle and enlargement of these may mimic disease in the gland.

Management Treatment is with antibiotics and excision of the stone perorally. If this cannot be achieved the whole gland may need to be removed by an external approach. Established infection may proceed to abscess formation.

Tumours

Fine needle aspiration of the mass should be performed. About 50% of tumours are benign, most commonly pleomorphic adenomas.

Management These should be excised with the entire gland, taking care to preserve the marginal mandibular branch of the facial nerve. Malignant tumours necessitate excision of the whole gland, with a radical neck dissection in certain cases.

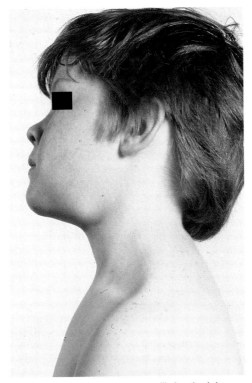

Fig. 141 Enlargement of the submandibular gland due to chronic infection.

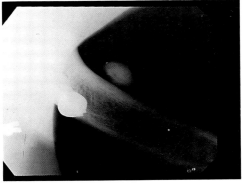

Fig. 142 Floor of mouth X-ray demonstrating a stone in the submandibular gland duct.

44 / Reconstruction in head and neck surgery

Following excision of a tumour from the head or neck, primary closure of a resultant tissue defect with preservation of adequate function may not be feasible or cosmetically acceptable. Only by the introduction of tissue from another site can a satisfactory result be achieved. Such tissue may be used to provide lining (reconstruction of an internal mucosal defect) or cover (reconstruction of a skin defect).

Techniques
- *Non-vascularised free grafts.* These depend on the recipient site for their blood supply. Include split skin, full thickness skin, dermis, nerve and bone grafts.
- *Pedicled skin.* May be random, with a non-specific blood supply, or axial, when the flap has a named arterial blood supply, e.g. deltopectoral flap (Fig. 144) and pectoralis major myocutaneous flap (Fig. 145).
- *Revascularised free grafts.* The artery and vein supplying the graft tissue are re-anastomosed to vessels at the recipient site. Include radial forearm flap (Fig. 143) and jejunum.
- *Pedicled viscera.* Stomach or colon may be used.

Several factors will determine the choice of flap/graft for the individual patient.

Myocutaneous flaps and re-vascularised free grafts have meant that the lining of an internal surface can be carried out as a one-stage procedure, greatly reducing hospitalisation time.

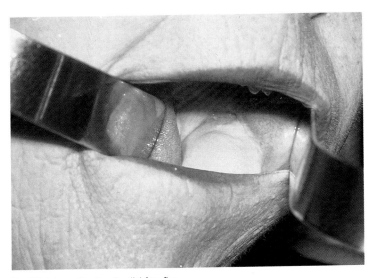

Fig. 143 Intra-orally placed radial free flap.

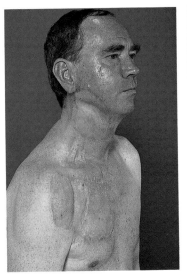

Fig. 144 Neck skin replacement using a deltopectoral flap.

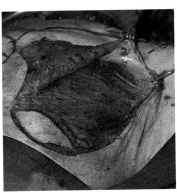

Fig. 145 Pectoralis major flap just prior to division of the muscles' attachments.

45 / Palsies of the last four cranial nerves

Aetiology   Often involved together by lesions in the brainstem or at the skull base, e.g. lateral medullary syndrome, CVA, motor neurone disease, glomus tumour, meningitis, nasopharyngeal carcinoma.

Glossopharyngeal nerve

This nerve is sensory to the posterior third of the tongue (including taste) and pharyngeal mucosa. Motor to middle constrictor.

Clinical features   It is rarely paralysed alone. A unilateral palsy does not produce severe functional disability.

Vagus nerve

This nerve is sensory to the larynx and motor to the soft palate, pharynx and larynx. Also sensorimotor to the thoraco-abdominal viscera.

Aetiology   An isolated palsy of the recurrent laryngeal branch is usually either idiopathic or due to disruption of the nerve in the neck or chest, e.g. post-thyroidectomy, bronchial carcinoma (Fig. 146).

Clinical features   Variable. Palatal paralysis, hoarseness, weak cough, overspill of food and secretions and airways obstruction may all occur, although a recurrent laryngeal nerve palsy will not produce palatal paralysis.

Management   Airway incompetence due to a unilateral cord palsy may be helped by injection of Teflon into the paracordal tissues to increase the cord's bulk (Fig. 147). Bilateral palsies may produce total airways obstruction or serious overspill. A tracheostomy will be required in either case.

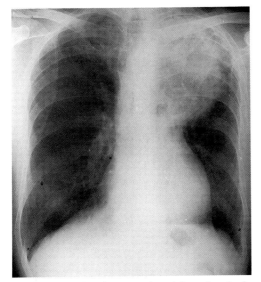

Fig. 146 Bronchial carcinoma causing a left vocal cord palsy.

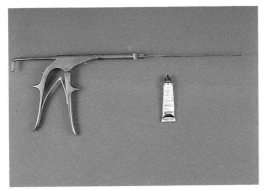

Fig. 147 Teflon gun for endoscopic injection of a paralysed vocal cord.

Accessory nerve

The spinal part of this nerve is motor to sternomastoid and trapezius. An isolated palsy is seen after a block dissection of neck or injudicious posterior triangle lymph node biopsy.

Clinical features The shoulder assumes a dropped appearance (Fig. 148) and the patient is unable to shrug or abduct the shoulder to a vertical position.

Management A resultant frozen shoulder may benefit from physiotherapy.

Hypoglossal nerve

This nerve is motor to tongue and hyoid depressors. An isolated palsy is usually iatrogenic, e.g. following laryngectomy or submandibular gland excision, or due to malignant disease in the upper neck.

Clinical features On protrusion the tongue deviates to the paralysed side (Fig. 149). Wasting and fasciculation indicate lower motor neurone damage. Unilateral palsies are usually asymptomatic. Bilateral palsies produce severe dysarthria and swallowing difficulties.

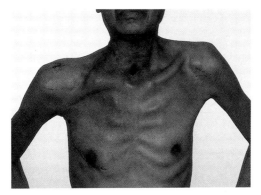

Fig. 148 Dropped shoulder following right neck dissection (and laryngectomy).

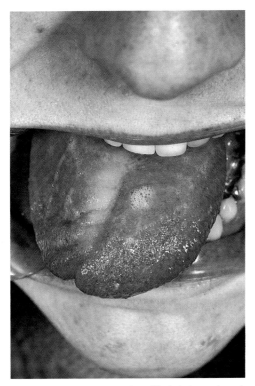

Fig. 149 Hypoglossal nerve palsy with deviation and wasting of hemitongue.

46 / Human immunodeficiency virus (HIV) infection

ENT manifestations of HIV infection commonly fall into one of three groups.

Cervical lymphadenopathy

Clinical features
Common. May be persistent generalised lymphadenopathy (PGL) or secondary to pharyngitis. However, rapidly enlarging, asymmetrical (Fig. 150) or fixed nodes may herald a lymphoma, Kaposi's sarcoma or an occult squamous carcinoma.

Management
In cases where malignancy requires exclusion, fine needle or open biopsy is necessary. The treatment will then depend on the pathological diagnosis.

Kaposi's sarcoma (KS)

The skin and mucosa of the head and neck are common sites for KS in AIDS patients.

Clinical features
Lesions present as red or purple macules, plaques or nodules. Palatal involvement is most common (Fig. 151). Rarely, KS may cause airway obstruction.

Management
Treatment is multi-modal.

Oral cavity 'hairy' leucoplakia

Clinical features
Leucoplakic patches on the lateral border and ventral surface of the tongue (Fig. 152) which have a tendency to regress and recur. Possibly caused by the Epstein-Barr virus (EBV). Microscopically the keratin whorls give a hairy appearance. The lesion should be distinguished from candidiasis, also common in these patients. Rapid progression to full blown AIDS is common once 'hairy' leucoplakia has developed.

Management
Treatment is by biopsy and observation of the lesion, whose malignant potential remains unknown.

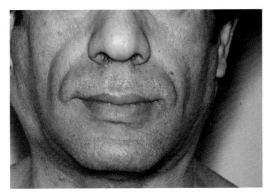

Fig. 150 Asymmetrical cervical lymphadenopathy in PGL.

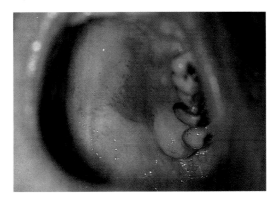

Fig. 151 Kaposi's sarcoma of the hard palate.

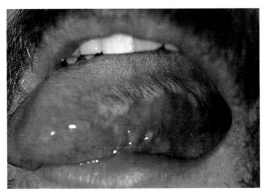

Fig. 152 Hairy leukoplakia of the lateral border of the tongue.

Index